HYPERTHYROIDISM DIET COOKBOOK

Easy-To-Follow Recipes For Reducing Symptoms, And Boosting Energy With Nutrient-Dense Meals

DR ELIAN GRIFFIN

DISCLAIMER

The nutritional recommendations and recipes in this book are meant solely for informative reasons. They are not meant to replace the counsel, diagnosis, or care of a qualified medical expert. If you have any doubts about a medical condition or dietary requirements, you should always see your physician or another trained healthcare expert.

All reasonable efforts have been taken by the author and publisher to ensure that the information contained in this book is correct as of the date of publication. Recommendations may alter, though, as medical knowledge is always changing. When using any of the recipes or instructions found here, the user assumes all liability and assumes no risk, whether personal or otherwise. People who have certain dietary requirements or medical issues should speak with a healthcare provider for personalized guidance. The given recipes are only ideas; you may need to adjust them to suit your own nutritional needs, tastes, and tolerances.

When you use this book, you agree to release the publisher, the author, and their representatives from any liability for any claims, damages, liabilities, costs, or expenditures resulting from your use of the book.

TABLE OF CONTENTS

ABOUT THE BOOK

The "Hyperthyroidism Diet Cookbook" is an indispensable tool for people attempting to manage their hyperthyroidism through food decisions. Comprehending the subtleties of hyperthyroidism is essential since it impacts metabolism and general well-being. The first section of this book defines hyperthyroidism, discusses its causes, and goes over potential symptoms. Crucially, it highlights how diet plays a part in controlling these symptoms and how important it is to have medical advice to customize food to meet specific health requirements.

Throughout the book, the significance of following a customized nutrition plan is emphasized. People with hyperthyroidism can maximize their dietary intake while reducing potential triggers that worsen symptoms by following a diet that is conducive to their condition. The cookbook offers precise recommendations for items to include and stay away from, guaranteeing a well-rounded approach to fulfilling dietary needs.

To support long-term health management, regular monitoring is emphasized as being crucial for tracking progress and modifying dietary plans accordingly.

With its layout designed to make practical use easier, this cookbook provides thorough meal planning and preparation methods. It gives readers the skills they need to easily incorporate nutritional changes into their daily lives, from efficient grocery shopping suggestions to batch cooking for maximum efficiency. The recommendations for necessary kitchen equipment are included to make sure readers are ready to easily complete the recipes.

The recipe sections are made to accommodate different dietary needs and meal times. There's enough protein for breakfast, a well-rounded lunch, and healthy dinner recipes to go along with tips for controlling portion sizes and adding some spice to the kitchen. Extra attention is paid to drinks, desserts, and snacks; they provide wholesome substitutes that enhance general health without sacrificing taste.

Aware of the variety of dietary requirements, the cookbook also offers recipes catered to certain food sensitivities and modifications for vegetarian, vegan, dairy-free, and gluten-free diets. This adaptability highlights the book's dedication to inclusivity by guaranteeing that people with different dietary limitations may still savor tasty and nourishing meals.

The book offers helpful guidance on negotiating social settings, dining out, and traveling while following a certain diet, as well as answers to frequently asked questions. It provides resources for further assistance and investigates substitute ingredients, enabling readers to uphold dietary observance and improve their quality of life.

"Hyperthyroidism Diet Cookbook" is a thorough manual that provides people with useful resources and mouthwatering recipes that help them efficiently control their hyperthyroidism through careful food selection.

CHAPTER ONE

HYPERTHYROIDISM DIET INTRODUCTION

KNOWING ABOUT DIET AND HYPERTHYROIDISM

The disorder known as hyperthyroidism occurs when the thyroid gland overproduces thyroid hormone, which interferes with metabolism and other body processes. In addition to pharmaceutical interventions, managing hyperthyroidism entails dietary modifications to promote general health and reduce symptoms. Because some foods can either help regulate thyroid function or exacerbate symptoms, it is important to understand the role that diet plays in this process. People with hyperthyroidism can better control their condition and enhance their quality of life by concentrating on a balanced diet designed specifically for managing the illness.

When following a diet for hyperthyroidism, one should prioritize foods that promote thyroid function and steer clear of those that could encourage the synthesis of excess hormones. Important nutrients for thyroid hormone synthesis and control are zinc, selenium, and iodine. Foods high in these nutrients, like dairy products, nuts, seeds, and seafood, may be advantageous. However, to avoid aggravating symptoms of hyperthyroidism, foods high in iodine, like seaweed and iodized salt, should be taken in moderation.

Not only does one need to know what to eat, but also how much and how often to eat it to manage hyperthyroidism. Meals that are smaller and more frequent can help control blood sugar levels and avoid increases in the production of thyroid hormone. It is essential to seek advice from a medical professional or a trained dietitian to customize a food plan that effectively manages hyperthyroidism while fulfilling personal demands and health objectives.

DIET IS CRUCIAL FOR MANAGING HYPERTHYROIDISM

Because some foods can either help or impede thyroid function, diet is important in managing hyperthyroidism. Those who suffer from hyperthyroidism may find that eating a balanced diet helps control thyroid hormone production and reduce symptoms including jitters, fast heartbeat, and weight loss. Through the adoption of a nutrient-dense diet that minimizes foods that may exacerbate symptoms, people may be able to decrease their reliance on medication and enhance their general health.

For hyperthyroidism, a well-balanced diet usually consists of fruits, vegetables, lean meats, and whole grains in various combinations. Essential vitamins, minerals, and antioxidants found in these foods promote immunological function and help sustain energy levels. Reducing intake of refined carbohydrates, sugar, and caffeine is also advised because these substances can aggravate symptoms of hyperthyroidism, such as anxiety and insomnia.

Knowing how nutrition affects thyroid function gives people the power to make decisions that will benefit their long-term health.

A person's quality of life can be improved and their condition can be better managed by including foods high in nutrients and avoiding triggers. Thyroid function is regularly monitored with blood tests, and diet modifications are made as necessary to keep dietary decisions in line with general health objectives and symptom management techniques.

ADVANTAGES OF A PARTICULAR DIET PLAN

For those who are treating hyperthyroidism, there are various advantages to adhering to a customized nutrition plan. An organized eating plan lowers symptoms including irritation, weight loss, and an accelerated heartbeat by regulating thyroid hormone levels. Focusing on meals high in nutrients that promote thyroid function may help people feel more in control of their mood, have more energy, and generally feel better.

A well-crafted hyperthyroid diet plan makes it clear which items are safe to eat and which should be avoided, making grocery shopping and meal planning easier.

This method eliminates uncertainty and guarantees that people regularly eat items that support thyroid function and lessen the exacerbation of symptoms. In addition, a regimented diet plan promotes following dietary recommendations, enabling people to actively participate in controlling their health and reaching their goals.

Following a prescribed food plan also helps people feel in charge of their health, which boosts motivation and self-assurance when it comes to controlling hyperthyroidism. People can support long-term health goals by embracing evidence-based dietary guidelines and tracking how these recommendations affect their thyroid function and symptoms.

Consultations with dietitians or healthcare professionals regularly guarantee continued assistance in the efficient management of hyperthyroidism and help tailor the food plan based on individual responses.

HOW YOU CAN USE THIS COOKBOOK TO HELP

This hyperthyroidism diet cookbook is intended to serve as a useful and educational tool for anyone considering using food to control their condition. It provides a selection of delectable and nourishing meal options along with a selection of dishes that are specially chosen to assist thyroid health. With components that are good for thyroid function included in every meal, people may maintain a balanced diet without compromising taste or variety.

This cookbook offers helpful insights into the fundamentals of a thyroid-supportive diet along with helpful meal preparation advice, in addition to recipes. It provides inventive methods to include nutrient-dense foods like lean proteins, entire grains, and vibrant veggies in regular meals while highlighting their significance. People can confidently navigate their food choices and properly control their hyperthyroidism by adhering to the recipes and advice offered.

The cookbook offers tools for additional knowledge and assistance, as well as a thorough explanation of how eating affects thyroid health. It empowers people to take control of their health and promotes a proactive approach to managing hyperthyroidism through a balanced diet. This cookbook provides helpful advice and delectable dishes to help you on your path to improved thyroid health, regardless of whether you're looking to improve your existing management approach or receive a new diagnosis.

A SUMMARY OF THE COOKBOOK FORMAT

The introduction to hyperthyroidism and its dietary implications is the first section of our user-friendly hyperthyroidism diet cookbook. Subsequently, it shifts into multiple recipe segments, with each segment concentrating on distinct meal types, including breakfasts, lunches, dinners, and snacks. Clear instructions, nutritional data, and suggestions for item replacements to suit dietary restrictions and personal tastes are included with every dish.

A section on meal planning and batch cooking is also included in the cookbook, providing tips and techniques for organizing the weekly preparation of thyroid-supportive meals. A special focus is on the procurement of ingredients, with suggestions for maximizing nutritional value by choosing locally and organically obtained foods whenever feasible. To ensure readers new to managing hyperthyroidism through dietary alterations have clarity and knowledge, the cookbook also includes a glossary of terms relating to hyperthyroidism and diet.

Overall, this cookbook's layout aims to empower people with hyperthyroidism to choose foods wisely and in line with their health objectives. This cookbook offers a complete resource to support your journey towards improved thyroid health via diet, whether you're looking for ideas for new meals or helpful tips on grocery shopping and meal preparation.

CHAPTER TWO

COMPREHENDING HYPERTHYROIDISM

OVERVIEW OF HYPERTHYROIDISM

The overproduction of thyroid hormones by the thyroid gland is the hallmark of hyperthyroidism. The body's metabolism may be greatly impacted by this imbalance, which may result in several symptoms like abrupt weight loss, an accelerated heartbeat, anxiety, and irritability. The thyroid gland, which is situated in the neck, produces hormones like triiodothyronine (T3) and thyroxine (T4) that are essential for controlling metabolism. Excess production of these hormones can speed up biological processes beyond normal limits, leading to hyperthyroidism.

Thyroid hormone and thyroid-stimulating hormone (TSH) levels are often measured by blood tests, and physical examinations are performed to evaluate symptoms and thyroid gland size. Depending on the severity, there are a variety of treatment options available, such as radioactive iodine therapy to shrink the thyroid gland, medicines to lower hormone production, or, in extreme situations, surgery to remove the thyroid gland entirely.

REASONS AND SIGNS

There are several causes of hyperthyroidism, but the most prevalent one is Graves' disease, an autoimmune condition in which antibodies cause the thyroid gland to overproduce hormones. Thyroid nodules or thyroid gland inflammation (thyroiditis) are additional possibilities.

Symptoms frequently start mildly and then get more severe over time, greatly affecting day-to-day living. Elevated heart rate, shaking palms, heat sensitivity, weight loss despite heightened appetite, and trouble sleeping are typical symptoms. Additionally, some people may exhibit emotional symptoms including anxiety, irritability, or mood swings.

Diet is essential for controlling hyperthyroidism symptoms since it promotes general health and may have an impact on thyroid function. Although there isn't a single diet that may treat hyperthyroidism, there are dietary approaches that can assist manage symptoms and promote thyroid function. Eating a balanced diet full of whole grains, fruits, vegetables, and lean proteins is crucial. Iodine-rich foods, such as shellfish and iodized salt, should be taken in moderation because too much of it can sometimes make hyperthyroidism worse.

Furthermore, abstaining from stimulants like alcohol and coffee may help control symptoms like anxiety and a fast heartbeat. Some people find that following an anti-inflammatory diet or cutting back on gluten helps reduce symptoms; nevertheless, these strategies should be explored with a healthcare professional. When making dietary adjustments, it's important to regularly check thyroid hormone levels because dietary modifications might not be enough to control the symptoms of hyperthyroidism.

THE VALUE OF MEDICAL ADVICE

For those who have been diagnosed with hyperthyroidism, seeking medical counsel is essential to creating a customized treatment strategy. Endocrinologists and primary care physicians, for example, can check thyroid hormone levels, offer advice on medication administration, and talk about possible therapy choices. In addition to medical care, they might suggest dietary modifications and stress-reduction strategies as lifestyle modifications.

To evaluate the efficacy of treatment and make necessary pharmaceutical adjustments, routine examinations, and monitoring are crucial. It's crucial to avoid self-diagnosing or self-treating hyperthyroidism since poor treatment might result in consequences like osteoporosis or cardiac issues. Working together with healthcare professionals guarantees that treatment programs are efficient, safe, and compliant with the most recent medical standards.

It's important to have reasonable expectations for how therapy will go and how symptoms will be managed when managing hyperthyroidism. Although thyroid hormone levels can be efficiently controlled by drugs or therapies, reaching optimal health may need patience and time. During treatment, it's common to have symptom variations or need to change the amount of your medications.

To manage hyperthyroidism realistically, one must acknowledge that it is frequently a lifelong process requiring constant monitoring and sometimes therapeutic modifications. Modifications to one's diet and methods of stress management are examples of lifestyle adjustments that can improve general health and manage symptoms. People can manage the difficulties of having hyperthyroidism by keeping lines of communication open with medical specialists, asking for help from medical experts, and joining support groups.

To properly manage hyperthyroidism, it is imperative to comprehend its causes, symptoms, the function of food, the significance of medical advice, and the need to set reasonable expectations. Over time, people with hyperthyroidism can improve their quality of life and attain improved health outcomes by managing their health proactively and working collaboratively with healthcare specialists.

CHAPTER THREE

THE ESSENTIAL DIET FOR HYPERTHYROIDISM

ESSENTIALS OF A DIET SUITABLE FOR HYPERTHYROIDISM

It's critical to prioritize nutrient-dense foods that support thyroid function when managing hyperthyroidism through diet while avoiding those that may increase symptoms. Maintaining a balanced diet of critical nutrients—like zinc, selenium, and iodine—is crucial for the generation and regulation of thyroid hormones. Thyroid health can be supported by including foods high in these nutrients, such as dairy products, nuts, seeds, and seafood. Furthermore, a diet high in whole grains, fruits, and vegetables provides antioxidants and fiber, which promote general health and help control hyperthyroidism-related symptoms including anxiety and weight loss.

Limiting stimulants like caffeine and refined carbohydrates is another important part of a hyperthyroidism-friendly diet, as these foods can exacerbate symptoms like agitation and palpitations. Choosing complex carbohydrates over simple sweets and herbal teas or decaffeinated beverages instead helps to balance mood and energy levels. Frequent, well-balanced meals spread out throughout the day can help control blood sugar levels and ward off energy slumps, which is especially advantageous for those whose hyperthyroidism causes higher metabolic rates. Following these fundamental guidelines can help people take control of their condition by making dietary decisions that promote healthy thyroid function and general well-being.

FOODS TO TAKE AND LEAVE OUT

Certain foods are essential for maintaining thyroid function in a hyperthyroidism diet, while others should be restricted or avoided to properly manage symptoms. Seaweed, salmon, dairy products, and eggs are among the foods high in iodine. This is because iodine is a component of thyroid hormones. Whole grains, seafood, and Brazil nuts are among the foods high in selenium that assist control of thyroid hormone synthesis and shield the gland from oxidative damage. Consuming these foods in moderation guarantees that the thyroid isn't overstimulated while getting enough nutrients.

On the other hand, excessive iodine from supplements and iodized salt should be avoided by those who have hyperthyroidism since it might worsen symptoms. Reducing processed food intake, which frequently has high sodium and refined sugar content, helps keep blood sugar stable and lowers inflammation. Broccoli, cabbage, and Brussels sprouts are examples of cruciferous vegetables. These vegetables should be cooked or eaten in moderation because they contain substances that, in high quantities, may interfere with the generation of thyroid hormone. People can effectively control the symptoms of hyperthyroidism and improve general health by paying attention to nutrient-rich, balanced meals and using mindfulness when making dietary decisions.

Since hyperthyroidism can alter metabolism and nutrient absorption, it is critical to balance dietary requirements when controlling the illness. Sufficient consumption of protein derived from lean foods such as fish, chicken, beans, and legumes promotes muscle growth and repair, which can be hampered in hyperthyroidism patients because of their elevated metabolic needs. Oily fish, flaxseeds, and walnuts are good sources of essential fatty acids that support cardiovascular health and reduce inflammation—important because hyperthyroidism can impair heart function.

A diversified diet that provides an adequate amount of vitamins and minerals is crucial for thyroid function and general health. Fortified dairy products and fatty fish are good sources of vitamin D, which helps maintain healthy bones and the immune system, both of which can be weakened in hyperthyroidism patients. B vitamins, especially B12, and folate, which are present in meat, dairy products, and leafy greens, enhance nerve function and energy production, which helps to reduce symptoms like anxiety and exhaustion. A balanced diet and a focus on nutrient-dense foods can help people improve their nutritional intake and support thyroid function and general wellness.

CONSISTENT MONITORING IS ESSENTIAL

When controlling hyperthyroidism with diet, it is crucial to regularly check nutritional status and thyroid function. Thyroid hormone levels can be monitored, usually with blood tests, to evaluate the impact of dietary modifications and, if necessary, prescription medication. Regular evaluation of nutritional status is also necessary to guarantee sufficient intake of vital nutrients including zinc, selenium, and iodine, which are critical for thyroid function.

Furthermore, keeping an eye on symptoms like energy fluctuations, weight changes, and heart rate swings offers insightful information about how well dietary plans work to manage hyperthyroidism.

Based on the results of the monitoring, the diet can be modified to better manage symptoms and improve general health. For example, nutrient-rich meals might be increased or decreased. Frequent consultations with medical professionals, such as endocrinologists or certified dietitians, guarantee thorough management of hyperthyroidism and offer direction on how to best customize food choices to meet personal needs and tastes.

EXAMPLE MENUS

For people with hyperthyroidism, a balanced diet plan should include meals high in nutrients and low in triggers that worsen symptoms. For breakfast, a normal day's menu can consist of Greek yogurt with berries and a handful of nuts for antioxidants and protein. A little apple with almond butter could be a mid-morning snack to provide prolonged energy and healthy fats.

A spinach salad with grilled chicken, avocado, and quinoa for lunch might provide a good mix of fiber, protein, and other important elements.

For extra protein and fullness, try an afternoon snack of mixed nuts or carrot sticks with hummus. Steamed broccoli and quinoa paired with baked salmon would be a healthy dinner option. The omega-3 fatty acids, fiber, and selenium in the salmon enhance thyroid function and general health.

Drinking water or herbal teas to stay hydrated throughout the day promotes general health and metabolism. Meal planning that prioritizes nutrient-dense foods and balances macronutrients helps people with hyperthyroidism efficiently manage their symptoms while promoting optimal thyroid function and general health.

CHAPTER FOUR

MEAL PLANNING AND PREPARATION

STRATEGIES FOR EFFICIENT MEAL PLANNING

To effectively manage a diet for hyperthyroidism, meal planning is necessary. To begin with, ascertain your nutritional needs and preferences. Make a weekly meal plan that includes breakfast, lunch, dinner, and snacks to start. Pay attention to nutrient-dense foods including lean meats, whole grains, and an abundance of fruits and vegetables that promote thyroid function. Take into account meal timing and amount sizes to keep your energy levels consistent throughout the day. To guarantee a balanced intake of vitamins and minerals, include variation.

Choosing dishes that are simple to make and freeze well is a sensible strategy. Make inventive use of leftovers to reduce waste and save time. Utilize applications and web resources that include grocery list capabilities and meal planning templates.

Adapt your menu to your particular preferences and the available food during the season. As you plan your meals, don't forget to include hydration and emphasize the importance of drinking water throughout the day.

TIPS FOR GROCERY SHOPPING

Effective food shopping is essential to keeping a diet that is suitable for hyperthyroidism. Make a thorough grocery list to start, depending on your food plan. Give lean meats, healthy grains, and fresh produce the top priority; steer clear of processed foods that are high in sugar and sodium.

Look for seasonal and fresh ingredients that promote thyroid health at your local farmers' markets. To save money and cut down on store visits, think about buying staples like grains and legumes in bulk.

When planning your shopping excursions, try to avoid the crowds and reduce your stress levels. Carefully read food labels to steer clear of any hidden additives that could make your hyperthyroid symptoms worse.

Whenever feasible, use organic products to minimize your exposure to hormones and pesticides. Your grocery list should be varied to keep things interesting and the nutrients balanced. Finally, for increased convenience—especially during hectic weeks—take into account online grocery delivery services.

COOKING IN BULK FOR OPTIMAL EFFICIENCY

A useful tactic for keeping to a restricted diet and streamlining meal preparation is batch cooking. Start by choosing meals that are easy to reheat and freeze well. Set aside a certain day of the week to cook in bulk, with an emphasis on preparing large amounts of food ahead of time. Use high-quality, microwave- and freezer-safe storage containers to help maintain food quality and make reheating easier.

Portion control and waste reduction can be achieved by dividing your batch-cooked meals into separate units. To guarantee freshness and simple identification, mark each container with the contents and the date of preparation.

Add adaptable ingredients that may be used in several dishes during the week, such as quinoa, legumes, and roasted veggies. To keep things interesting and avoid meal fatigue, switch up your batch-cooking recipes. As necessary, adjust the tastes and seasonings to your taste.

ESSENTIAL KITCHEN TOOLS AND EQUIPMENT

Meal preparation for a hyperthyroid diet can be streamlined by stocking your kitchen with the necessities. When preparing meals, start with high-quality knives and cutting boards to ensure safety and effectiveness.

Invest in a food processor or blender to make soups and smoothies that are loaded with ingredients that are high in nutrients. For hands-off cooking of stews and grains that maintain their nutritional value, try using an Instant Pot or slow cooker.

Make sure you have enough measuring spoons and cups in your kitchen so you can portion ingredients precisely as per your meal plan.

Reduce the amount of additional fats and oils required for cooking by using non-stick cookware. To make handling a variety of dishes easier, include utensils such as ladles, tongs, and spatulas.

To guarantee safe food handling procedures, maintain kitchen hygiene using dish towels, sponges, and cleaning products.

SETTING UP YOUR MEAL PLAN

The secret to keeping your hyperthyroidism diet balanced and consistent is to plan your meals. To start, allocate some time each week to prepare meals according to your nutritional needs and timetable. Plan your daily meals for breakfast, lunch, dinner, and snacks using a calendar or meal planning software. During hectic workdays, think about meal prepping in bulk to save time and lower stress.

Set up a space in your kitchen for meal preparation and label clear storage containers to keep food storage neat and orderly.

To make sure you have all the ingredients on hand, plan your meals around your supermarket shopping excursions. As your schedule or impending events change, make the necessary adjustments to your food plan. Schedule wiggle room for impromptu dinners or occasions when you want to eat out but still adhere to a healthy, balanced diet.

IDEAS FOR HEALTHY AND EFFICIENT BREAKFASTS

Here are some quick and healthy breakfast alternatives that fit within a hyperthyroidism diet to help you start your mornings off right. Think about choices like antioxidant-rich smoothie bowls with nutrients that assist the thyroid. For a nutrient-rich and refreshing breakfast, blend spinach, berries, chia seeds, and a dairy-free milk substitute.

A quinoa breakfast dish with roasted veggies and a scattering of pumpkin seeds for extra protein and important minerals is an additional choice.

Overnight oats are a godsend for people who are always on the go. The night before, make them with almond milk, gluten-free oats, and garnishes of almonds, seeds, and a little honey for sweetness. These oats give you steady energy throughout the morning and are quite customizable. Finally, try avocado toast on gluten-free bread topped with hemp seeds and a squeeze of lemon.

Avocado is a great option for a balanced breakfast because it delivers good fats that support thyroid function.

RECIPES PACKED WITH VITAL NUTRIENTS

Examine breakfast recipes that are rich in nutrients that are critical for thyroid health maintenance. For a protein boost, start with an omelet packed with veggies and cooked with eggs or egg whites. For a vibrant and nutrient-dense lunch, add bell peppers, tomatoes, and spinach. For a full breakfast, serve with a slice of gluten-free bread.

Try a tofu scramble seasoned with black pepper and turmeric for an anti-inflammatory plant-based option. For extra fiber and vitamins, try tossing tofu with sautéed greens like collard or kale. Tofu is a fantastic source of protein. A Greek yogurt parfait packed with fresh berries, almonds, and seeds is another nutrient-dense choice. Probiotics included in Greek yogurt help maintain gut health, which is crucial for thyroid function as a whole.

A REVIVING BEGINING TO YOUR DAY

Start your day off right with a nutritious breakfast that supports thyroid function and fuels your body. Start with a protein powder or nut butter scoop for extra energy and satisfaction, a banana for sweetness, and a bowl of leafy greens like spinach or kale for maximum nutrition. Smoothies made with spinach are high in vitamins and minerals and easy to digest.

As an alternative, consider having a modest amount of sweet potatoes or steamed veggies together with a lean protein source like turkey or chicken sausage. Protein aids in blood sugar stabilization, which is advantageous for hyperthyroid individuals. A whole grain breakfast bowl with brown rice or quinoa, topped with avocado, roasted veggies, and a poached egg for protein and good fats, is another satisfying choice.

ADVICE FOR HECTIC MORNINGS

It's essential to prepare for hectic mornings. Think about preparing breakfast items in bulk, such as veggie- and lean-protein-packed egg muffins. These are a convenient grab-and-go food that can be prepared in advance and kept in the freezer or refrigerator. Another easy breakfast option that requires no work in the morning is overnight oats or chia seed pudding made in individual jars.

On the weekend, prepare items for your meals and organize your kitchen to set yourself up for success. This guarantees that you always have wholesome breakfast options on hand and saves time during the workweek. If you're often on the move and need to pack breakfast for your commute to work or your trip to the gym, consider investing in bento boxes or portable containers.

TIPS FOR PREPARING MORNING MEALS

Master the art of preparing breakfast with useful advice that will make your morning routine easier. Plan your breakfast for the upcoming week first. Pick dishes that can be prepared ahead of time, including baked oatmeal squares with fruit and nuts on top, overnight oats, and breakfast burritos with whole-grain wrappers.

Wash and cut veggies, portion out dry ingredients (like quinoa or oats), and cook meats (like turkey sausage or hard-boiled eggs) ahead of time to save time when preparing ingredients. To preserve freshness, store prepared components in meal prep or sealed containers.

Use your freezer to prepare large quantities of foods that can be swiftly reheated in the morning, such as muffins or breakfast sandwiches. For simple identification, mark containers with the contents and dates. Finally, to make your morning routine run more smoothly, schedule a fixed time each week for preparing breakfast. This will guarantee that you begin each day with a filling and healthy meal that is appropriate for your hyperthyroidism diet.

LUNCH OPTIONS THAT ARE SATISFYING AND BALANCED

Choosing a meal that is both balanced and filling is essential for diet-based hyperthyroidism management. A combination of lean proteins, complex carbohydrates, healthy fats, and an abundance of veggies should ideally make up a balanced lunch. Begin with a foundation of nutritious grains, such as brown rice or quinoa, which offer fiber and long-lasting energy. To enhance the health and metabolism of your muscles, combine this with lean proteins like beans, tofu, or grilled chicken breast. Incorporate wholesome fats such as avocado or olive oil to promote thyroid function and satiety.

For vital vitamins, minerals, and antioxidants, a good chunk of your meal should consist of vegetables. Choose a colorful variety that is high in nutrients and fiber, such as broccoli, bell peppers, carrots, and leafy greens. Including a balanced lunch promotes general well-being by guaranteeing you receive a variety of nutrients necessary for optimum health, in addition to helping to manage the symptoms of hyperthyroidism.

SIMPLE LUNCH IDEAS TO PACK

Easy-to-pack lunch ideas make meal preparation simpler and help you keep to your hyperthyroidism diet if you lead a busy lifestyle. Choose to make meals in advance and store them in handy containers. A healthy and portable option is salads made out of a variety of leafy greens, cherry tomatoes, cucumbers, and a lean protein source, such as grilled salmon or chickpeas. For a nutritious lunch on the run, whole grain wraps stuffed with hummus, sliced tofu or turkey, and fresh veggies are another option.

Another great option is soup, which can be prepared in large quantities and frozen in individual servings for simple reheating. For a hearty and nutrient-dense lunch, choose homemade soups that are loaded with veggies and lean meats like chicken or lentils. In addition to saving you time, these quick lunch alternatives make sure you're giving your body the essential nutrients to promote thyroid function.

Including meals high in fiber and antioxidants can help manage the symptoms of hyperthyroidism and promote general wellness. Antioxidants can be especially helpful for those with thyroid disorders as they shield the body from oxidative damage and inflammation. To increase your consumption of antioxidants, incorporate foods like berries, nuts, seeds, and dark leafy greens into your lunch meals.

In addition to being vital for maintaining healthy digestion, fiber also plays a key role in blood sugar regulation for those with hyperthyroidism. To boost fiber content, base your lunch meals on whole grains like quinoa, barley, or oats. Additionally, great providers of fiber and legumes like beans and lentils can be added to salads, soups, or grain bowls for a filling and healthy lunch alternative.

When organizing lunches for people with hyperthyroidism, controlling portion sizes is essential. Consuming meals that are well-balanced and with sensible portion sizes aids in controlling energy levels and metabolism all day long. Try to have half of your plate composed of veggies, 25% of it composed of lean proteins, and 25% of it composed of nutritious grains or complex carbohydrates.

Steer clear of excessive servings of high-calorie foods that might cause weight gain and worsen the symptoms of hyperthyroidism.

Rather, prioritize nutrient-dense foods that offer vital vitamins and minerals without being overly caloric. You can better control the symptoms of hyperthyroidism and maintain a healthy weight by properly controlling portion sizes.

Adding diversity to your meals not only adds enjoyment to mealtimes but also guarantees that you receive a wide range of nutrients that are essential for thyroid health. To vary your nutrient intake, try rotating your sources of lean proteins, such as fish, poultry, tofu, or beans. To keep meals exciting and nutrient-dense, try experimenting with different whole grains, such as quinoa, brown rice, or whole wheat pasta.

To optimize nutrient diversity, pack your lunches with a rainbow of veggies. Different vitamins, minerals, and antioxidants that are good for general health are available in each color group. To spice up your meals and make sure you're eating what's on your plate, experiment with different dishes and cuisines. You may keep up a balanced diet that promotes thyroid function and general well-being by mixing up your lunches.

DINNERS THAT ARE NOURISHING FOR OPTIMAL HEALTH

Choosing ingredients rich in critical nutrients and balancing flavors for a satisfying meal are key components of preparing nourishing dinners that support optimal health while managing hyperthyroidism. Make sure to include lean proteins such as fish, poultry, or chicken since they contain the amino acids needed for hormone balance and muscle repair. Serve them with a range of vibrant vegetables, like broccoli, bell peppers, and leafy greens, which provide vitamins, minerals, and antioxidants essential for thyroid health.

Consider adding herbs and spices like turmeric, ginger, and cilantro, which not only provide depth but also have anti-inflammatory qualities, to boost flavor without depending too much on salt or high-fat components. By including healthy grains like brown rice or quinoa, you can avoid the energy dumps that are frequently linked to hyperthyroidism by consuming complex carbs that help maintain blood sugar levels. You may make dinners that support thyroid health and longer-lasting energy by emphasizing nutrient-dense foods and well-balanced meals.

ONE-POT DINNERS FOR EASE

One-pot meals are convenient and nutritious for people who manage hyperthyroidism. These dishes maximize nutrition and flavor while requiring the least amount of cleaning. To begin, choose a lean protein source, like beans or lean meat cuts, and then mix in a range of veggies, like tomatoes, spinach, and carrots. Use whole grains like barley or farro to provide you with long-lasting energy and fiber, which helps with digestion and blood sugar regulation.

When all components are cooked in one pot, the tastes combine and the nutrients are retained. To add flavor without adding too much salt, use homemade stocks or low-sodium broths as a foundation. To add richness and depth, play around with different herbs and spices like paprika, thyme, and rosemary.

One-pot meals are perfect for busy people controlling hyperthyroidism since they not only expedite the cooking process but also guarantee that each serving is balanced with important nutrients.

RECIPES WITH FEW TRIGGERING SUBSTANCES

Foods that can worsen symptoms must often be avoided to manage hyperthyroidism. When developing dinner meals, give special attention to foods low in triggers like gluten, processed sugars, and iodine. Choose fresh produce and fruits, such as kale, mushrooms, and apples that are naturally low in iodine. Select lean proteins, such as tofu or chicken, which supply essential amino acids without adding extra fats or salts.

Steer clear of prepackaged foods and make your dressings and sauces with basic ingredients like lemon juice, olive oil, and herbs. Making meals from scratch gives you more control over the ingredients and allows you to modify recipes to fit certain dietary requirements. To avoid gluten while still providing texture and taste, try baking with alternative flour like coconut or almond flour. You may make dinner recipes that are easy on the thyroid and promote general health by emphasizing whole, minimally processed foods.

COOKING METHODS FOR NUTRITION AND TASTE

Cooking methods that maximize flavor and retain nutrients must be mastered to prepare excellent meals while controlling hyperthyroidism. To preserve the natural flavors and nutrients of veggies, try roasting or steam-baking them. While roasting carrots or sweet potatoes caramelizes their natural sugars and intensifies flavor, steaming broccoli or cauliflower preserves their crisp texture and nutrient content.

For protein, consider baking or grilling fish or fowl with as little extra fat as possible. These techniques offer a light smokey flavor without compromising the integrity of the proteins. Try marinating meats in mixtures of herbs, garlic, and citrus liquids to impart flavor and tenderness without using a lot of salt or oil.

Dinner options for the whole family that are appropriate for people with hyperthyroidism must strike a balance between dietary requirements and palate-pleasing ingredients. Add adaptable components to your recipes, such as beans (a good source of fiber and protein) or pasta salads. Vegetables that are good for kids, such as bell peppers and zucchini, can be a smooth complement to other ingredients in stir-fries or casseroles.

To accommodate varying nutritional choices within the family, provide a variety of options, such as vegetarian dishes like vegetable stir-fry with tofu or grain bowls with quinoa and roasted vegetables. Allow kids to help with basic food preparation duties like stirring or garnishing, or let them select items. You may promote healthy eating practices and make sure that everyone at the table enjoys their meals by incorporating interactive and inclusive dinnertime activities.

TIPS FOR HEALTHY SNACKING

It is essential to keep a balanced diet when managing hyperthyroidism. Snacking healthily is essential for maintaining energy levels and promoting general well-being. Choose snacks that are low in harmful fats and carbohydrates and high in nutrients including vitamins, minerals, and fiber. Because they are low in calories and high in antioxidants, fresh fruits and vegetables are great options. For a filling and healthy snack, think about options like carrot sticks with hummus or apple slices with nut butter. Furthermore, complex carbs included in whole grains like oats and whole wheat crackers assist in balancing blood sugar levels, preventing energy surges and crashes.

Add lean protein sources to your snacks, such as Greek yogurt or cottage cheese, to increase their nutritious content. These proteins support a healthy metabolism by aiding in muscle maintenance and repair. Because of their filling protein level and heart-healthy fats, nuts and seeds are especially useful. But keep in mind that these are high in calories, so watch your portion sizes. By eating consciously and without interruptions, you may pay attention to your hunger signals and truly enjoy and appreciate your food. By doing this, you can improve your digestion and avoid overindulging.

HEALTHY SNACK SELECTIONS

Selecting wholesome snacks that complement your hyperthyroidism diet entails emphasizing nutrient-dense foods that maintain flavor. Choose foods that are high in antioxidants, vitamins, and minerals—essential nutrients.

A handful of mixed nuts has protein and good fats that help with satiety and blood sugar regulation. Berries on top of Greek yogurt not only quell a sweet tooth but also provide gut health benefits from probiotics and immune system support from antioxidants. Try a small portion of low-fat cheese or whole-grain crackers with avocado slices for a savory option.

Because they are high in water content and fiber, fresh fruits and vegetables are a great option for maintaining regular digestion and staying hydrated. For a cool, nutrient-rich snack, graze on cucumber slices sprinkled with lemon juice or a vibrant fruit salad. Including whole grains increases the amount of complex carbs that provide you energy all day long. Examples of these include air-popped popcorn and whole wheat toast with almond butter. By providing you with sustained energy and satisfaction in between meals, these choices not only help maintain the health of your thyroid but also improve your general well-being.

RICH DESSERTS THAT ARE GOOD FOR YOU

Selecting desserts that are both decadent and health-promoting is essential while treating hyperthyroidism. Choose treats produced with natural sweeteners like maple syrup or honey instead of processed sugars, which cause a sharp jump in blood sugar levels while offering a rich flavor. Fruits such as bananas or berries give natural sweetness to sweets as well as fiber, vitamins, and minerals. For a filling and healthy dessert option, try a yogurt parfait made with layers of Greek yogurt, fresh berries, and honey drizzled over.

Try out these dishes using dark chocolate, which is well-known for its mood-enhancing and antioxidant qualities. A handful of almonds and a tiny piece of dark chocolate combine to create a tasty yet healthful dessert. If you're a baker, try looking for recipes that call for whole-grain flour rather than refined white flour, such as almond or oat flour. These substitutes achieve the desired texture and flavor while providing more nutrients and fiber. You can enjoy sweets that promote thyroid health and overall well-being by choosing carefully and striking a balance between enjoyment and nutritional content.

STRATEGIES FOR PORTION CONTROL

Maintaining a healthy weight and controlling hyperthyroidism need effective portion control. To visually fool your mind into feeling content with fewer servings, start by utilizing smaller dishes and plates.

Broccoli and other non-starchy veggies, which are high in fiber and minerals but low in calories, should make up half of your plate. Aim for a portion size that fits in your palm when serving protein-rich foods like fish or lean meats. By doing this, you can be sure you're maintaining your muscle mass without consuming too many calories.

Practice mindful eating techniques, such as chewing carefully and appreciating each bite, to prevent thoughtless eating. Take note of your body's signals of hunger and fullness to avoid overindulging. To keep quantities under control, measure snacks and sweets rather than eating straight from the packet. For convenient grab-and-go solutions, choose single-serving packages or divide bigger servings into smaller containers. Making meal and snack plans in advance can also help with portion control because it will guarantee that you have the right serving sizes on hand for when hunger strikes. You may support the health of your thyroid by employing these measures to manage portion sizes and maintain a balanced diet.

Effectively controlling desires is essential when adhering to a hyperthyroidism diet to preserve optimum health and well-being. Recognize the distinction between cravings brought on by emotions or habits and actual hunger. When a craving hits, take a little stroll or engage in another activity to divert your attention and prevent yourself from indulging in an impulsive snack. Determine the factors that cause cravings, such as stress or exhaustion, and come up with alternate strategies to deal with these feelings, including learning relaxation techniques or getting enough sleep.

Select nutrient-dense foods that will help you achieve your health objectives while satisfying cravings. If you're craving something sweet, try a small piece of dark chocolate or a bowl of fresh fruit with some Greek yogurt on top. Grab some air-popped popcorn seasoned with herbs or a handful of mildly salted nuts to satisfy your cravings for something savory. To lessen temptation, hide harmful snacks and swap them out for healthier options. When enjoying goodies, exercise moderation and take your time, savoring each bite instead of scarfing them down. You may effectively manage cravings and maintain a balanced diet to support thyroid health by recognizing your cravings and putting good coping methods into practice.

WATER AND ITS FUNCTION IN THE MANAGEMENT OF HYPERTHYROIDISM

By sustaining general physiological processes and fostering thyroid health, hydration is essential for the management of hyperthyroidism. Drinking enough water aids in controlling body temperature and metabolism, both of which hyperthyroidism patients may have abnormalities in. It also helps with electrolyte balance maintenance and toxin removal, both of which are critical for healthy muscle and neuron function.

Maintaining adequate hydration levels for people with hyperthyroidism requires more than simply drinking water; it also entails making sure that electrolyte balance is maintained and consuming fluids that promote thyroid function. Because an imbalance in thyroid hormone can impact nerve and muscle function, electrolytes like potassium and magnesium are especially crucial. Consuming foods high in water content, such as cucumber, watermelon, and coconut water, can also help maintain electrolyte balance and general hydration.

Aim for at least 8 to 10 glasses of water each day to be well-hydrated, and adapt as necessary depending on your personal activity level and the surroundings. In addition to promoting hydration, herbal teas, and infused water can be great options for adding diversity and taste. These drinks can support a hyperthyroidism diet by providing extra health advantages in addition to fluids.

THE ADVANTAGES OF HERBAL TEAS

Herbal teas can boost thyroid function and general health, making them ideal complements to a diet for hyperthyroidism. Some herbs, such as motherwort, lemon balm, and bugleweed, are well known for their ability to soothe the thyroid gland and lessen the overproduction of thyroid hormones. Additionally, they have antioxidant qualities that can shield cells from harm brought on by free radicals, which is advantageous for those who have hyperthyroidism.

It's critical to select caffeine-free herbal teas when introducing them into your diet, as caffeine may aggravate hyperthyroidism symptoms. In addition to being hydrating, herbal teas with relaxing properties like chamomile and peppermint can aid with anxiety reduction and sleep improvement—problems that are frequently linked to hyperthyroidism.

Herbal teas can be made by steeping 1-2 tablespoons of dry herbs in 5–10 minutes of hot water, depending on the strength that is desired. Pour through a strainer and serve warm or cold, with the option to add stevia or honey for natural sweetness. You can maximize the health advantages of your daily hydration regimen by experimenting with different herbal mixtures.

JUICES AND SMOOTHIES TO BOOST NUTRIENTS

Juices and smoothies are easy ways to increase nutritional consumption and promote general health, particularly for those who are controlling hyperthyroidism. They offer a concentrated form of antioxidants, vitamins, and minerals that can boost immune system health and fight oxidative stress, which is especially advantageous in cases of thyroid dysfunction.

Nutrient-dense components that promote thyroid health can be added to smoothies and juices, such as leafy greens, berries, flax seeds, and coconut water. Vitamin C-rich foods like oranges and strawberries can assist enhance the absorption of iron, which is important because iron deficiency can lead to nutritional shortages.

Blend a variety of fruits, veggies, and liquids (such as almond milk or coconut water) to produce nutrient-dense smoothies.

 Supplementing protein sources, such as Greek yogurt or protein powder, can improve nutritional value and help maintain muscle mass. Fresh fruit and vegetable juices have additional health benefits, but it's important to drink them in moderation to prevent consuming too much sugar.

For people with hyperthyroidism, limiting coffee consumption is essential since it might stimulate the nervous system and perhaps aggravate symptoms including palpitations, anxiety, and insomnia. As part of a hyperthyroidism diet, caffeine should be limited or avoided because it can also affect thyroid function and hormone synthesis.

Decaffeinated coffee, herbal teas, and caffeine-free sodas are some examples of caffeine-free options that can help cut down on caffeine use without sacrificing enjoyment or hydration. It's critical to carefully check labels because even beverages that are advertised as caffeine-free occasionally contain traces of the stimulant.

If you appreciate the ritual of making coffee or tea, cutting back on caffeine gradually and switching to herbal substitutes might lessen withdrawal symptoms and promote general well-being. Without depending on coffee, staying hydrated throughout the day with water and herbal infusions can also assist sustain energy levels and promote metabolic function.

INNOVATIVE AND COOL DRINK CONCEPTS

Even when controlling hyperthyroidism, staying hydrated can be fun and varied with the exploration of inventive and refreshing drink alternatives. Slicing citrus fruits, cucumbers, or mint leaves into water to infuse not only improves flavor but also provides vital vitamins and minerals that promote general health.

Another hydrated choice is coconut water, which also contains electrolytes like magnesium and potassium, which are essential for healthy muscles and nerves.

Fresh fruit juices and sparkling water combined to make mocktails can enhance hydration and nutritional intake while offering a festive substitute for alcoholic beverages. Herbs like rosemary or basil can bring reviving flavors to beverages as well as extra health advantages like support for the digestive system and anti-inflammatory properties.

Try making homemade iced teas with cold-brewed green tea or caffeine-free herbal mixes for a pleasant drink that boosts antioxidants and hydration. In addition to being hydrating, smoothie bowls with fresh fruit, nuts, and seeds on top provide a filling and healthy snack that can be tailored to each person's taste preferences.

You can improve your daily routine's hydration, promote thyroid health, and enjoy a wide variety of flavors and nutrients by including several inventive and refreshing drink ideas. These are all crucial elements of a diet for hyperthyroidism.

CHAPTER FIVE

OPTIONS FREE OF DAIRY AND GLUTEN

Adopting a gluten- and dairy-free diet can help people with hyperthyroidism manage their symptoms and maintain overall health. Wheat, barley, and rye include gluten, which can occasionally cause inflammation and digestive problems that could worsen hyperthyroidism symptoms. For many people, dairy products—especially those with high lactose content—can potentially aggravate inflammation and digestive problems. People can lessen possible triggers and improve gut health by removing these from their diets.

Focusing on naturally gluten-free grains like quinoa, rice, and maize is crucial for successfully navigating a gluten-free and dairy-free diet since they offer vital nutrients without exacerbating symptoms. Dairy substitutes like cashew cheese, almond milk, and coconut yogurt can help keep calcium levels stable without having the inflammatory effects of regular dairy products. A varied and satisfying diet is ensured by investigating dishes that inventively replace dairy and gluten-containing components. This strategy improves digestion and lowers inflammation, which benefits thyroid health while also enhancing general well-being.

VEGAN AND VEGETARIAN RECIPES

When controlling hyperthyroidism, switching to a vegetarian or vegan diet can have several positive effects on your health, such as decreased inflammation and increased nutritional intake. Vegan diets forgo all animal products, while vegetarian diets remove meat but allow dairy and eggs. Plant-based foods high in antioxidants, vitamins, and minerals necessary for thyroid function and general health are the focus of both diets. Eating plenty of fruits, vegetables, legumes, nuts, and seeds guarantees a varied nutrient intake that promotes thyroid health and general well-being.

Tofu, tempeh, lentils, and chickpeas are just a few examples of plant-based protein sources that can be used to create balanced, fulfilling vegetarian and vegan dishes. Essential amino acids are provided by these components, which are critical for the immune system and muscle maintenance in hyperthyroidism patients. Playing around with different herbs, spices, and sauces improves the nutritional content and flavor of food, which makes it more pleasurable and healthy. People can enjoy a variety of delectable vegetarian and vegan meals while maintaining optimal thyroid health by focusing on natural foods and nutrient-dense components.

RECIPES FOR CERTAIN ALLERGIES TO FOODS

Careful meal planning is necessary while managing food allergies and hyperthyroidism to prevent symptoms from getting worse and aggravating existing medical conditions. Allergies to common foods such as eggs, shellfish, peanuts, and tree nuts can range in severity from minor discomfort to life-threatening respiratory distress. For those with hyperthyroidism, creating recipes that eliminate allergenic components without sacrificing nutritional balance is crucial. Making use of safe and nutrient-dense substitute components guarantees that meals are satisfying and promote general health.

Creating recipes for people with particular food sensitivities requires exchanging allergenic items with safe substitutes. For example, nut and gluten allergies can be accommodated by using sunflower seed butter instead of peanut butter or coconut flour instead of wheat flour. Adding freshly squeezed lemon juice, herbs, and spices amplifies flavor without depending on common allergens. One way to maintain a diet that supports thyroid health and lowers the likelihood of allergic reactions is to avoid pre-packaged items that may contain hidden allergens and instead concentrate on eating whole, unprocessed foods.

CUSTOMIZING RECIPES TO FIT PERSONAL TASTES

People with hyperthyroidism can tailor their diets to suit their tastes while still making sure they are getting enough nutrients.

Customization is essential to sustaining long-term dietary adherence and general well-being, whether it is done by modifying recipes to suit taste preferences, dietary constraints, or health objectives. Individuals can improve thyroid health and overall quality of life by preparing meals that are both nourishing and pleasant by experimenting with different foods, cooking techniques, and portion sizes.

Understanding dietary needs and preferences is necessary when customizing recipes to suit individual preferences. For instance, you can accommodate particular dietary requirements and preferences by changing the cooking methods, replacing certain products, or reducing the amount of flavor. Including a range of tastes and textures makes meals enjoyable and fulfilling, which encourages dietary compliance and improves general health. People can maintain a balanced diet that promotes thyroid function and improves overall well-being by embracing culinary creativity and flexibility.

For those with hyperthyroidism, modifying diet regimens is essential to maximizing dietary intake, controlling symptoms, and advancing general health. Since each person has different dietary requirements and preferences, customized meal plans that target particular health issues and objectives are required. Through customization of diet regimens to incorporate foods high in nutrients, maintain a balance in macronutrient intake, and account for personal sensitivities or allergies, people can improve their quality of life and support thyroid function.

Understanding the value of personalization entails working with medical experts to create dietary plans that satisfy both individual preferences and medical guidelines. Placing a strong emphasis on whole foods, lean proteins, healthful fats, and complex carbohydrates guarantees a balanced diet that promotes metabolic and energy wellness.

CHAPTER SIX

FREQUENTLY ASKED QUESTIONS

TAKING CARE OF DIETARY RESTRICTIONS

To maintain optimal health when managing a hyperthyroidism diet, food limits must be addressed. Your health can be greatly affected by knowing which foods to prioritize and which to avoid. Iodine-rich foods such as seafood, iodized salt, and dairy products should be avoided or consumed in moderation at first since too much iodine might aggravate symptoms of hyperthyroidism. Rather, concentrate on including nutrient-dense foods like whole grains, fruits, vegetables, and lean proteins. These options assist thyroid function generally in addition to supplying necessary vitamins and minerals.

Managing dietary limits also means keeping an eye on the items that cause goiter, which can cause disruptions in the production of thyroid hormones. Among these are cruciferous foods, such as Brussels sprouts, cauliflower, and broccoli. When these veggies are cooked, their goitrogenic effects are lessened, making them safer to eat in moderation. Thyroid abnormalities can also be made worse by stimulants like caffeine and processed foods that are heavy in sugar and trans fat. You can enhance the health of your thyroid and more effectively manage your dietary restrictions by giving complete, unprocessed foods and mindful eating habits priority.

It takes organization and ingenuity to incorporate dietary restrictions into your daily life, particularly when dining out or going to social events. To get ready, check out the menus online and let the servers or cooks know any dietary restrictions you have.

To limit your intake of iodine and goitrogen, choose plain, grilled foods and request dressings and sauces on the side. When you socialize, remember that it's more important to enjoy the company than the food. To make sure you have options, bring a dish or snack that complies with your diet.

You may maintain the health of your thyroid and confidently handle social situations by taking proactive measures to manage dietary constraints.

MANAGING SOCIAL MEDIA AND DINING OUT

When following a hyperthyroidism diet, navigating social settings and dining out calls for careful preparation and communication. Notifying loved ones of your dietary limitations will help you feel less stressed and make sure you have appropriate options available. When dining out, study the menus ahead of time and select items that meet your needs, like salads without high-iodine components like dairy or shellfish, or grilled proteins and steamed veggies. Tell the staff at the restaurant about your tastes; they will often be able to fulfill unique requests or substitute ingredients.

Pacing yourself throughout meals and paying attention to portion quantities are other important aspects of handling social situations. Rather than feeling compelled to eat something that might not be good for your thyroid health, concentrate on enjoying the company and conversation. If you have dietary restrictions, think about bringing a dish to share so you have something to eat. To make sure your meal satisfies your dietary requirements, don't be afraid to ask questions if you have any doubts regarding the contents or the preparation process.

You may enjoy social gatherings and stick to your hyperthyroidism diet at the same time by being proactive about social situations and eating out.

ADVICE FOR PASSENGERS ON A SPECIAL DIET

To preserve your health and well-being when traveling on a particular diet for hyperthyroidism, you need to be prepared and adaptable. To find items that meet your dietary requirements, start by investigating the local food scene and grocery stores in your travel destination. Store non-perishable snacks like dried fruits, almonds, and seeds in your bag so you always have something to eat between meals and on the go. For perishable goods that might not be easily accessible, such as fresh produce, yogurt, and fruits, think about packing a tiny cooler or an insulated bag.

When dining while traveling, be sure to let the restaurant staff know about any dietary restrictions you may have, and when possible, request tailored selections. To steer clear of unidentified sources of iodine or goitrogens, opt for straightforward, lightly processed foods like grilled meats, steamed veggies, and rice or potatoes. Drink lots of water and herbal teas to stay hydrated. Avoid alcohol and caffeine, as they might interfere with thyroid function. You may properly manage your hyperthyroidism diet and yet enjoy travel by being proactive about your dietary demands and making advance plans.

INVESTIGATING SUBSTITUTE INGREDIENTS

Investigating substitute components for a hyperthyroid diet will increase your gastronomic alternatives while promoting thyroid function. To limit iodine intake, switch out iodized salt with non-iodized types or occasionally use sea salt.

Try experimenting with anti-inflammatory herbs and spices such as turmeric, ginger, and cinnamon, which may also have positive effects on thyroid function. Instead of using vegetable oils heavy in omega-6 fatty acids, which can exacerbate inflammation and thyroid imbalance, use avocado or olive oil.

Using non-dairy milk alternatives, such as almond, coconut, or oat milk, in place of cow's milk in dishes and drinks is another way to incorporate alternative ingredients. Frequently enhanced with vitamins and minerals, these substitutes maintain flavor and texture when used in baking and cooking. Seaweed or kelp flakes can be used in smoothies, salads, and soups as a natural, regulated source of iodine. You can improve the nutrient density and thyroid health of your meals by experimenting with different flavors and component combinations.

LOOKING FOR RESOURCES AND ASSISTANCE

Staying informed and motivated on your path to health requires looking for assistance and resources for managing a hyperthyroidism diet. Make contact with medical specialists who specialize in thyroid health, such as registered dietitians or endocrinologists, who can offer individualized supervision and guidance. Participate in internet forums or support groups devoted to thyroid diseases to exchange stories, pose inquiries, and gain insight from individuals with comparable dietary difficulties.

Investigate reliable sources of information about diets for hyperthyroidism as well, such as books, websites, and instructional materials from reliable medical associations. Keep abreast with developments in thyroid health research so that you may make well-informed choices regarding your lifestyle and food. If you want to learn more about thyroid function and nutrition and expand your knowledge of these topics, consider attending seminars or workshops. You might learn new techniques for properly managing your health.

www.ingramcontent.com/pod-product-compliance
Lightning Source LLC
Chambersburg PA
CBHW061301250726

48653CB00002B/728